FATMAP
STUDY GUIDE

Getting Off Autopilot

GERALD KEITH JACKSON

Fulton Books
Meadville, PA

Published by Fulton Books 2024

Cover Design: Gerald K. Jackson
Cover Design Assistant: Tosha R. Jackson

FATMAP Study Guide is not medical advice and is not intended as treatment for any illness or medical disease. This study guide does not offer exercise programs, recipes, or radical diets. It focuses on a much deeper wellness dilemma.

ISBN 979-8-89221-173-4 (paperback)
ISBN 979-8-89221-174-1 (digital)

Printed in the United States of America

Gerald Jackson,

You have enriched many lives through your publications. You have inspired over five thousand subscribers each month with your expertise. That is why I've personally selected you as the only fitness writer for *Epitome Magazine*.

Be blessed,
Todrick Johnson, publisher
Epitome Magazine

CONTENTS

Introduction...vii
Overview..ix

Mindset
    Lesson 1:   Acknowledging Your Attitude..............................3
    Lesson 2:   Language and Attitude 5
    Lesson 3:   Facts about Food Analysis 8
Meals
    Lesson 4:   Speaking to Your Body 13
    Lesson 5:   Control.. 15
    Lesson 6:   Eating by the Clock, Not by the Calendar.......... 16
Movement
    Lesson 7:   Always Do Something.. 23
    Lesson 8:   Good Health Is Earned, Not Purchased 25
    Lesson 9:   Moving Toward Your Goal 27
Motive
    Lesson 10: What Is Your Why? 33
    Lesson 11: Goals versus Results.. 36
    Lesson 12: Gratitude.. 38

From the Author 41
Notes and Analysis Review 43
    Physical Activity Readiness Questionnaire (PAR-Q)............44
    FATMAP Step-by-Step Helpful Tips 45
    Keys to Success..45
Resources 49

INTRODUCTION

The most basic objective of life is not to preserve youthfulness. The first rule is to preserve self.

My *FATMAP Study Guide* will not help you discover the fountain of youth. Rather, this book will teach you how to start and maintain a successful health and fitness journey. My goal is to show you how to live a healthy, prosperous life of longevity and fulfillment!

OVERVIEW

Good health starts with winning the battle
against your own free will.

Have you ever wondered why there is a demand for personal fitness trainers, diet plans, dietitians, nutritionists, and life coaches?

Ever wondered why people intentionally make unhealthy food choices when healthier foods are an option? The answer is "free will." Unfortunately, your free will is not freedom if you behave as a prisoner of unhealthy habits. Neuroscience research suggests your brain does not differentiate between good and bad habits. According to Dr. Norman Doidge, habits are just habits!

Therefore, the fight against unhealthy choices is really a fight against your personal nature. The good news is, winning the battle for better health really comes down to a choice that only you can make.

My *FATMAP Study Guide* focuses on more than diet and exercise. It delves into your mindset, motive, and attitude about health. This powerful triad serves as the main pillars of your success or failure!

If you're interested in improving your health, but can't seem to get out of your own way, my *FATMAP Study Guide* is for you! Follow along and I will break down many years of health and wellness research into four simple categories:

- Mindset
- Meals
- Movement
- Motive

Mindset

Acknowledging Your Attitude

I've witnessed unhealthy people struggle to become healthier because they lacked a healthy *mindset*. What do I mean by mindset? Your attitude about health, in general, and how you prioritize eating and exercise is a mindset. If you are still unclear about assessing your mindset, look at it this way, your *mindset* is demonstrated by your daily habits!

Mindset also includes self-perception. I'm not referring to the person in your mirror. I'm talking about the person in your mind. Who is that?

- Who is the person inside of your brain?
- What is your perception of you?
- How accurate is that perception?

The person looking at you in the mirror is the physical manifestation of how you've been treating yourself.

How others see you is predicated on what you show them! For this reason, it is important to surround yourself with people who inspire you to elevate your well-being.

Who is your inspiration? I'm talking about the person who prompts you to check your attitude about your health? What energizes you to reach beyond your comfort zone toward becoming better? How often do you engage with individuals who inspire positive change in your life? I'm not referring to those who allow you to simply talk the talk. I'm looking for the one who holds you accountable to walk the walk!

Acknowledging the influence of your social circle along with your daily habits is the first conversation you must have. Before you can gain control and achieve better results, you have to first acknowledge how you really behave when it comes to certain thoughts and acquaintances, then we'll focus on prioritizing food and exercise.

The quickest and easiest way to notice your eating habits is to go into your kitchen and open your pantry. Is your pantry filled with instant foods to include sweet and salty snacks? Open the kitchen drawers. Are your kitchen drawers filled with condiments with fast-food logos on them? Finally, check inside of your car and office desk. Do you see bags or receipts from restaurants? If so, there's your answer!

My experience revealed one thing all people have in common: no one chooses to live with poor health!

LESSON 2

Language and Attitude

The following information is not intended to be overly technical.

By simply following the process used by my most successful clients, you will discover how changing your language will "help get your mind right."

My message is simple—give purpose to your meals and movement!

I had a client who did not accept my "eat less to weigh less" philosophy. At that time, she exercised four days per week. She freely ate without restrictions. Her goal was to lose weight; instead, she gained twenty unwanted pounds!

After that, I refused to train her in my gym for one month. During her time away from the gym, she made better food choices and lost twelve pounds without exercising!

If you are like most people, *diet* is a bad four-letter word. I was told that if you remove the letter *T* from the word *diet*, it spells *die*!

The word *diet* is derived from the Greek word *diaita*, which means "way of life." Think about it for a moment. Your way of life encompasses much more than counting calories and cutting out your favorite food. Your way of life includes:

- Education
- Occupation
- Income
- Belief system
- Social status and more

The word *diet* has less to do with food and more to do with your way of life. Is your way of life conducive for good health?

Continuing to focus on language brings me to the most overly utilized word in the fitness industry—sacrifice!

This is how it sounds: "I guess I can sacrifice giving up my chips and cookies!" Giving up something you don't need and something that is not good for you is *not* a sacrifice!

Other language barriers pertaining consumption are innocent terms like *breakfast*, *lunch*, and *dinner*.

The word *breakfast* triggers a desire for foods you may need to avoid.

For example, the word *breakfast* makes you think of:

- pancakes
- biscuits
- syrup
- butter
- doughnuts
- pastries
- pork sausage
- dairy milk
- waffles
- toasted bread
- jellies and
- jams

The word *lunch* triggers a different urge for foods like:

- hamburgers,
- French fries,
- onion rings,
- pizza,
- hot dogs,
- chili dogs,
- corn dogs,
- chili cheese nachos,

- grilled cheese sandwiches,
- sugary soft drinks,
- high-calorie dairy shakes, and
- cakes and pies,

The following items trigger cravings from the word *snack*:

- salty chips
- sweet pastries
- sugary cookies
- cupcakes
- twinkies
- hard candies
- candy bars

LESSON 3

Facts about Food Analysis

Imagine a drop-down menu descending from inside of your brain whenever you hear words such as *breakfast, lunch, dinner,* or *snack*. Replace those words with:

- Meal 1
- Meal 2
- Meal 3, etc.

All meals should resemble a healthy dinner plate. If the most important meal of the day is breakfast, shouldn't it also be the healthiest meal?

What are a few things people can't live without?

The answers are *oxygen, sunlight,* and *water*. Oxygen, sunlight, and water should be a part of your food intake. How can you eat sunlight and oxygen? Simply look for foods that require sunlight and oxygen to grow. Yes, I'm talking about real food! The human body has thrived on real food since the beginning of time.

It wasn't until people started overly consuming foods not found in nature that America experienced an obesity epidemic for the first time in recorded history!

Food that does not require oxygen, sunlight and water are manufactured artificially. This can cause metabolic problems due to the lack of natural ingredients. A diet consisting of mostly unnatural foods interfere with your digestive process, and the food chemicals affect your mind. Food addiction is really chemical addiction.

Remember, focus on developing a successful mindset first. This will help you strengthen healthier habits and weaken, or possibly eliminate unhealthy habits.

Keys to a Successful Mindset:

- Focus on what you can eat.
- Do not focus on foods you are giving up.
- Prepare meals one to two days ahead.
- Use natural seasonings such as peppers and onions.
- Store healthier food in convenient, portable containers to avoid making unhealthy choices.

Incidentally, an obesity epidemic does not fall from outer space, nor is it caused by the slowing down of your metabolism. The average person has no idea what a word like *metabolism* means. Just remember, metabolism is every chemical process happening in your body! It is unlikely you will be able to accurately measure the speed of your metabolism with any instrument. Stop worrying about the speed of your metabolism. Instead, start moving, make healthier food choices, and let your metabolism do the rest!

Exercise, from the medieval Latin term *practica*, means "to practice."

Conclusion: Proper diet and exercise simply means practicing a proper way of life conducive to good health!

Meals

LESSON 4

Speaking to Your Body

When I first started my personal training business, I heard people say things like "calories in, calories out, right?" I said no! It's not calories in, calories out. All calories are not useful. Calories are like words. There is such a thing as empty calories just as there are empty, meaningless words. Here's what I mean.

If your car's gas tank can hold a maximum of twenty gallons of fuel, what would happen if you filled the gas tank with twenty gallons of syrup? Would the engine fire? Would the car start? Would your car benefit? Of course not! More than that, you are causing major damage to the motor by feeding it something it was not designed to run on. You filled your gas tank with empty calories. Empty calories have zero positive effect!

Learn to speak your body's language! Tell your body what to do by feeding it what it needs, and stop eating useless calories.

Feeding your body to lose weight is not about how little you eat, rather, how much you eat!

Your body interprets ingredients, calories, vitamins, electrolytes, minerals, nutrients, proteins, carbohydrates, fats, and water. It also responds to glucose, sodium, iron, potassium, and other metabolic fuel.

Based on how you feed it, your body gains or loses weight, energy, muscle, fat, etc.

A perfect example of this is witnessed in the sport of boxing. Body weight is critical in the boxing circuit, because a boxer's weight determines competition eligibility. From boxing, I discovered I did not have to change my exercise regimen to lose or gain weight. I only had to change my eating!

Feeding your body enough food to lose unwanted pounds is simply the opposite of feeding your body enough to gain a desired weight. It's not about gaining or losing weight. It's all about weight control! I will discuss control in more detail in lesson 5.

Note: The right foods create the right internal environment. For example, eating fresh fruit, vegetables, and lean protein while avoiding junk food, fast food, alcohol, and trips to vending machines allows your body to lose unwanted weight and body-fat.

Doubling or tripling your calories tells your body to keep packing on the pounds!

LESSON 5

Control

Why is it risky to eat anything you did not prepare?

You have no control over how it was prepared. You have no idea how much salt or sugar was used. This means you have no control over calories.

The idea for better health is that you stop depending on someone else to feed you!

If you have to eat a hamburger, cook it yourself! If you have to eat fried chicken, find a healthier way to fry it!

There was a time when everything was homemade. People ate lots of good food made at home. Before vending machines, fast food, and twenty-four-hour restaurants, there was no report of an obesity epidemic.

People rarely ate away from home in the 1960s and 1970s. Practically every meal was prepared at home, where adults *controlled* how food was prepared.

These days, parents are not ashamed to confess their children will not eat anything other than popular fast-food restaurants that offers French fries daily!

In the 1960s and 1970s, the majority of adults did not have gym memberships. They weren't on fad diets, yet they were lean! Want proof? Look at TV shows and movies from the 1960s and compare them to today's movie body types. What changed?

Eating by the Clock, Not by the Calendar

If you've ever been around someone with a newborn baby, you will hear the phrase "It's *time* to feed the baby." Newborn babies eat on schedule.

Eating by the clock creates a routine for when to eat, but more importantly, for when *not* to eat. Eating *by* the clock prevents you from eating *around* the clock!

I ask these three questions about healthy eating:

1. What food item are you eating?
2. How much of that item are you eating?
3. How often do you eat that much of that item?

Let's start with the *what*.

Overlook the marketing image on the product and focus on what your body sees. Your body sees ingredients! Your eyes see an ice cold glass of a refreshing, colorful drink. Yummy for your tummy, right?

However, your body sees artificial chemicals, food coloring, and table sugar.

What about the foods with labels containing words you can't pronounce?

The Food and Drug Administration (FDA) is doing their part by providing a label, but outside of the picture, you have no idea what you are putting in your mouth. Anything you put in your mouth affects your bloodstream and your brain. Depending on what it is, how much you consume, and how often you eat it, you can generate cravings for the ingredients.

Again, food addiction is really chemical addiction. People report craving products that are either sweet or salty. No one has ever reported craving spinach or being addicted to apples and fresh garden salad.

Real food should not contain a list of extra craving-causing chemicals on a label. For example, broccoli is broccoli, and cabbage is cabbage. When other stuff gets added such as sugar, artificial colors and flavors, the ingredients listed on the label gets longer. The label reads from left to right, with the most prominent ingredients listed first. Remember, your body has to sort out everything listed on that label.

Losing weight starts with regular daily trips to the restroom to eliminate waste, dispelling what would otherwise stay in your body indefinitely.

Phase 1 of my FATMAP program is called the *Elimination Phase*.

In phase 1, the primary objective is to speed up digestion. Speed up digestion by:

- Eating foods that are less dense in calories
- Avoiding highly processed foods

Another component of my FATMAP program is insulin response reduction. This is accomplished by eating low glycemic foods. It's okay if you are not familiar with the glycemic index. In short, the glycemic index measures the rise of your blood glucose after food consumption. The glycemic index ranges from zero to one hundred, where seventy and above is considered high. For more information, enter glycemic index in your search engine.

Here is a simpler explanation of blood sugar and insulin levels. Imagine attending a big festival with thousands of other event goers in Las Vegas, Nevada.

You arrive at your hotel, grab your luggage, and go inside the hotel lobby. Once inside, you make your way to the front desk. Before you get to the front desk, you have to wait in a line of crowded guests who booked the same hotel as you.

You finally get checked-in, and you are handed your room key. Now let's grab the luggage and make it over to the elevators before everyone else! Your room is on the twelfth floor. You wait patiently as others are exiting the elevator at a snails pace. You finally reach your floor. The elevator doors open. You walk through the corridors until you get to your room. Your magnetic room key does not unlock the door. You are stuck in the hallway with other guests experiencing the same problem. You eventually learn the hotel is overbooked and someone else is already occupying your room. What a bummer!

Here's the translation:

a. The hotel is your body.
b. The hotel lobby entrance is your mouth.
c. The hotel guests are sugar molecules.
d. The sugar molecules enters from your mouth into your body.
e. The front desk is your pancreas.
f. The room key is an insulin protein that attaches to the sugar molecule.
g. The key escorts you (the sugar molecule) to your room.
h. The hotel rooms represent cells in your body.
i. The elevators and hallways represent your bloodstream.
j. The room key is intended to grant the glucose molecule inside access to the room.
k. If your cells are already occupied by sugar molecules, access will be denied.
l. A rise in sugar and insulin remain in your bloodstream (the hotel hallway).
m. Hallways containing high blood-sugar and high insulin levels is the type 2 diabetes recipe.

Do not overbook your hotel! Focus on low glycemic foods to prevent this unhealthy chain of events.

Feed the muscle lean protein and amino acids. Consume low glycemic and low acidic foods. Create your food plan, and do not let your calendar influence your food selection.

How does the calendar influence food choices? Let's start with the first day of the year.

- New Year's Day – Celebratory food and alcohol in January
- Valentines Day – Chocolate and wine in February
- St. Patrick's Day – Fried food and Beer in March
- Easter – Restaurant dinner in April
- Mother's Day and Memorial Day – restaurant and cook-out in May
- Father's Day and Juneteenth – Cookout in June
- Independence Day – Cookout in July
- Football season – Tailgate food and alcohol in August
- Labor Day – Cookout
- Halloween – Candies and sweet snacks
- Thanksgiving – Big dinner, desserts, and spirits in November
- Holiday Spreads – Cakes, pies, and alcohol in December

This list does not include birthdays, anniversaries, weddings, company potlucks, weekend excursions, or any other reason to consume extra calories!

There's nothing wrong with participating in your favorite traditions, but you must protect the gift of good health! The attributes of good health are:

- Brighter outlook
- Think more clearly
- Better sleep
- Body fat reduction
- Strength
- Energy

- Stamina
- Strong immune system
- Healthy weight

Below are nine initiatives toward eating for good health:

- Bodily toxicity reduction
- Insulin response reduction
- Harmful food awareness
- Sustainable, healthier diet
- Speed up digestion
- Generate energy
- Strengthened immune system
- Reduced body-fat weight
- Improved mobility

Improving mobility brings us to my lesson about movement.

Movement

LESSON 7

Always Do Something

I stayed in shape for the following reasons:

- Independence
- Response to an emergency situation
- Peace of mind and self-confidence

For me, working out has never been about sex appeal! It's always been about responsibility. I can honestly say, "I've done my part to be at my best!"

EXERCISE RULE #1:

Don't start exercising by going all out! First, prepare your body with low-intensity movement.

You will benefit most by slowly progressing your level of intensity with appropriate modifications to safely build strength and stamina.

- Spend time working on range of motion.
- Avoid ballistic movements and risky weightlifting exercises.
- Gain control of your balance and flexibility.
- Basic core strengthening is important because your strength is generated from your center.

My definition for exercise is:

- Exercise is a specific movement throughout a predetermined range of motion that follows aligned patterns from start to finish.
- Exercise movements occur over a designated period of seconds and minutes.
- Exercise is repetitive, measurable, and progressive over gradually higher intensities.

Remember, good health is a lifelong practice. Being in shape is like discipline and being faithful. You are, until you're not!

Good Health Is Earned, Not Purchased

As a newly certified personal trainer, I realized that without direction and accountability, people are not going to consistently exercise on their own. In all my years as a trainer, I've never heard anyone say, "I like to exercise!"

However, I noticed people were pretty good about keeping scheduled appointments. I'm sharing this because if you treat your exercise schedule as if it were an important appointment, you would have a stronger commitment to exercising regularly. Getting regular workouts is mostly about being held accountable for staying on schedule. No excuses!

I began noticing how nothing got in the way of my clients' workout schedule. They literally put everything and everybody else on hold until their fifty-minute training session with me was over.

Advice can be given away, but your workout results aren't free! You still have to do the work regardless of what it takes!

I am a stickler for detail, and I specialize in teaching proper workout posture, body positioning, form, and technique. Workout posture is as critical during a workout as it is during a ballet performance. Good workout posture increases fluidity in movement and reduces potential injury.

When I look at the gym floor, in my head I see a workout grid. The workout grid helps me determine everything from foot placement to proper joint alignment. This imaginary grid inspired me to design a workout floor mat called the FATMAP. I received a U.S. patent for its design in 2021.

The FATMAP taught clients the perfect workout form so well that if they went to a different gym or a different trainer, they could tell if something was not correct.

There are countless benefits to exercise:

- Strength increase
- More stamina
- Blood oxygen increase
- Muscle development
- Improved balance

The only thing that exercise does *not* directly affect is your weight!

LESSON 9

Moving Toward Your Goal

Before putting on your running shoes, take some time to understand three types of goals:

- Immediate goals
- Ultimate goals
- Long-term goals

Your immediate goal is usually simple to figure out. Let's say you want to see the number on your weighing scale go down a few numbers the next time you check your weight. There's a big difference between a goal and a result.

You may think your goal is to lose a few pounds, but losing weight is not a goal; losing weight is a result. "Changing your eating habits is the real goal which will result in losing weight."

When people don't see the "right" number on the weigh scale, they immediately get discouraged, dissatisfied, disappointed, and distracted from the real goal.

Knowing what to change is goal number 1!

How are ultimate goals different from long-term goals?

Please do not confuse your ultimate goals with your long-term goals. There's a big difference. Here's what I mean.

When I was seventeen years old, my desire was to build muscle. I was 6'2" tall, 165 pounds. My desire was to achieve a weight of 200 pounds while maintaining 6 percent bodyfat, with a waistline of 32 inches.

In order to do this, I had to gain over 30 pounds of lean muscle and no body fat. I was able to reach my ultimate body composition goal of 200 pounds while maintaining 6 percent body fat, and a 32-inch waist.

This is important because it's not about gaining weight. My goal was to build muscle, and the result was 200 pounds on the scale. The scale does not know who's standing on it. Meaning, I could weigh 200 pounds at 22 percent body fat, (which, for a male is medically unhealthy), or I could weigh 200 pounds with less than 10 percent body-fat. Again, do not focus on weight. Focus on body composition.

My ultimate strength goal was to bench-press 300-plus pounds. At that time, the rule was, if you possess the ability to bench-press 100 pounds over your body weight, you would qualify among elite weightlifters. Again, this is merely an example to help you differentiate your ultimate goals from your long-term goals.

An example of my long-term goal was to be able to enjoy performing my favorite exercises with relative ease well beyond age 50.

I wanted to be strong, agile, quick, and healthy enough to continue doing much of the same workouts I've become accustomed to for more than twenty years.

To this point, I've never been hospitalized or diagnosed for having any illness requiring prescription medications.

Avoiding hospitals and prescription medications was another one of my long-term goals!

As for my body composition and strength, my long-term goal is to stay lean and strong. At the time of this project, my weight is a lean 185 pounds, a 32-inch waist, and I work out with 250 pounds on my bench press.

Your ultimate goal should be much different than your long-term goal. Either way, be relentless and unwavering. When setting your goal, be reasonable and not unrealistic.

We've discussed movement and goals, and this is where the rubber meets the proverbial road. None of your goals will be achieved without maintaining a proper food log!

Your food log tells you everything you need to know and where to make changes.

Write down everything you eat for at least ten days without changing your eating habits. Be honest, accept the truth, and be accurate. Those ten days can really serve as an eye-opener!

In 2005, I gave a fitness seminar in Grand Prairie, Texas. A woman stood up and told me, "I don't have to write down what I eat. I can just tell you what I eat." The woman appeared to be in her early forties. I replied, "Respectfully, you might be able to remember the color of the dress you wore to your high school prom, but you can't tell me one thing you ate two weeks ago Thursday." The lady quietly sat down as I continued my presentation.

Most people eat without awareness:

- No awareness of when they are eating
- Unaware of what they've already eaten
- Oblivious to what they might eat next

I explained that people are not wired to accurately recall what they've eaten no more than they are able to track their spending from memory.

In that same seminar, a woman stood up and said, "Well, I don't eat burgers, fries, and potato chips. And I don't drink sodas." Mind you, this woman was visibly about 60 to 80 pounds overweight.

My response to her was this: "I understand that you do not eat those items. If you don't eat it, it can't hurt you. Let's focus your attention on what you are eating." That's why we start with the food log.

Read the very next line slowly.

Don't trust anyone to tell you what to eat if they don't know what you eat!

This is what the food log is for!

One final note on the importance of your written food log. I've witnessed a woman who successfully lost forty unwanted pounds by accurately keeping her food log. After reaching her weight loss goal, she thought she'd no longer need my services. She told me she made a choice to continue her fitness journey without me, and she went her own way for a few months only to return after gaining the weight back.

I suggested for her to update her food log for the next ten days. She told me that she didn't want to keep her food log anymore, so I politely, but promptly refunded her money.

Not keeping the food log is *not* an option. If you are serious about getting good results, it is the most important thing you can do.

Now that I've explained the importance of keeping your food log, let's look at another element for good health.

It is encouraged by medical and fitness professionals to get proper nourishment through natural foods. But if you aren't able to get the right amount of nutrients, vitamins, protein etc., it is recommended that you try natural supplements that are formulated in a laboratory that is regulated by the Food and Drug Administration (FDA).

Supplements are 100 percent optional. If you need an example of the supplements I've used over the past ten years, feel free to visit myj42.com

Let's review what we've learned so far.

1. Mindset
2. Attitude
3. Language
4. Meals
5. Movement
6. Goals
7. Food log
8. Supplementation
9. Professional assistance

Motive

What Is Your Why?

When it comes to health, the most important thing is not diet and exercise—it's *mindset* and *motive*!

You should already know that good health is a gift!

It is a gift because everyone is not born with good health. Valuing this gift means being grateful for the gift of good health. Do not take for granted that your health is automatically maintained.

Show appreciation by taking care of your mind and body. Focus on healthy thoughts, foods, and activities. Avoid negative thoughts by avoiding conversations with people that promote negativity.

Look at it this way - Everything you put into thought is on your mind, and everything you put in your mouth is in your bloodstream. Thoughts are tangible energy vibrations that affect your body's chemistry on some level. If you don't believe me, think about the physical effects of a stressful thought!

Obviously, anything that flows through your bloodstream affects your brain. In your brain lives the pilot of your life's plane. The question is, who's flying your life's plane?

Imagine if you were an actual plane.

1. Your feet and legs are the landing gear.
2. Your torso is the fuselage.
3. Your arms and hands are wings.
4. Your heart is the plane's engine.
5. Your lungs are the exhaust system.
6. Your blood is the fuel.

7. Your head is the cockpit.
8. Your brain is the dashboard.

Can you tell me what's missing from the plane?

Review the list of eight items and see if you can figure out number 9. While you're figuring out what's missing, here's another question.

Have you ever wondered why some people can stay focused on health goals to include losing weight while others seem to struggle?

Now that we have the entire plane assembled, what do you think is missing from the plane?

If your answer is, 'The pilot is missing,' you are *correct*!

The pilot represents the more than hundred billion estimated neurological connections and activities that occur inside your brain daily.

Some psychologists refer to this network as your consciousness. Your consciousness allows you to process information as you navigate and negotiate real-life situations and scenarios.

What if I told you that you are not your body and you are not your brain?

Your consciousness tells your brain what to think and tells your brain what to tell your body to do. Simply stated, your brain and body do not respond to situations when you are unconscious! Get it? Without consciousness, your brain and body is like a jet plane without a pilot!

Those neurological connections and activities form a sensational nebula of miraculous neurological interactions that make you who you really are!

In layman's terms, you (the *pilot*) tell your brain what's important. You tell your brain what to remember and what to learn. Your brain, hands, voice, eyes, ears, and feet are simply tools. You however, are *not* your brain, and you are *not* your body. Your brain and body should be subservient to your instructions. As you learn, develop, and mature, you should be able to use your brain more effectively.

I use the airplane reference because the plane cannot leave the runway without the pilot!

This brings me to my bigger point. People who struggle with reaching health goals are stuck on autopilot!

By allowing their perceived circumstances to navigate the plane, they never reach their destination in a timely manner, if at all.

The time has come for you to get off autopilot and take control of your health. Get back inside of the cockpit and regain control of the plane!

Here's the connection. Planes don't get hijacked—pilots get hijacked!

Instead of focusing on calories, place your focus on food chemicals. All those food chemicals hijack the way you think!

Unhealthy habits are influenced and strengthened by stimulating chemicals entering your bloodstream and passing through your brain, causing you to unconsciously make decisions that are not healthy.

These chemicals throw you off course. Once off course, you either struggle to reach your destination, you never reach the destination, or you completely lose control of your plane and crash!

The solution is awareness of what those artificial additives and stimulants do to you.

Food chemicals are not only unnatural, but they cloud your ability to make healthier decisions.

The real question is, why is maintaining good health important to you? What is your reason?

Getting into your favorite outfit may not be a strong enough motive to keep you focused.

If your motive is weak, your effort will be weak!

Your success depends on an unrelenting, unapologetic *why*!

Your *why* is your energy, your force field and grit! Your why keeps you holding on and bouncing back! Your why is the reason you can't give up.

There's no army, law, or amount of money that can knock you off your why, so get an awesome why, and you can't lose!

If you do not have a powerful reason, I offer this. Time is the greatest opponent of all. Time is undefeated. Time is unforgiving. We are all given the same twenty-four hours to choose healthier options toward a better quality of life.

LESSON 11

Goals versus Results

Focus on your goal, and results will follow.

If you are still somewhat confused about what to do and how to eat, I offer the Six Components to Better Health!

Let's begin with simple terminology. Health refers to how you are physically and mentally functioning. Your general health is typically based on the following information:

- Blood pressure
- Heart rate
- Breathing and respiration
- Body temperature
- Eye, ear, nose, and throat check
- Abdominal area
- Questions about health concerns

There are limitless medical tests and assessments that your doctor can perform during a traditional annual physical examination. Depending on your medical history and current health status, some medical examinations are more thorough than others.

However, medical examination results do not reveal anything about your fitness level. People have walked away from medical assessments with major undiscovered health problems. Some are often given a clean bill of health but are completely out of shape! This begs the question, Can you truly be healthy if you are not fit?

Are you able to climb a flight of stairs without experiencing shortness of breath? If your answer is no, and you have no medical issues, this should be your motive to get fit!

LESSON 12

Gratitude

Life is about making memories, so you might as well make some good ones. When all you have left are your memories, they should put a smile on your face!

Remember this: your greatest opponent will always be the element of time, meaning, at some point, our memories will outlive us all, and time will remain undefeated.

For this reason, don't forget three simple rules: *Do something meaningful, memorable, and fun!* Value the gift of good health while you have time. When the going gets tough, your ability to persevere is tied to your faith, beliefs, and purpose in life.

Imagine if you were a Christmas tree. The star topping you is the crown representing your legacy. Will memories of you inspire others?

Your tensile of passion should wrap itself around your efforts from top to bottom.

The many strings of lights indicate the number of times you brought hope to someone you'd never met.

The ornaments of your attitude should be decked in positivity, persistence, faith, enthusiasm, gratitude, and humility.

The base of your tree is thoroughly wrapped with the blanket of your discovered interests.

Where you stand sits the gifts prepared for many. These gifts are to be shared.

Among the many gifts are three larger gift boxes belonging to you. Inside the three larger gift boxes are the gifts of life, health, and strength. The better you nurture the three larger gifts, the better you can enjoy sharing the rest of them.

Inside one of those gift boxes, you will find your purpose.

Look at your reflection in a nearby glass. Does it look like you took your time and focused on the details before you're on display?

Or does it look as though you procrastinated until the eleventh hour before begrudgingly throwing it all together?

Are you that Christmas tree displaying a lack of investment of time and effort in yourself?

Every single prickly needle on your branches represent the number of hours you put into personal growth and self-development toward your purpose.

If you've taken advantage of the time you've been given, your branches would now be full, luminous, and far reaching!

No matter the case, don't ever stop carving out the details of your life. Look it over carefully. Look up and down the tree until you find a spot that's empty.

Once you discover a branch that's bare, adorn it with trinkets of meaningfulness.

With a little help, you will be decked to completion. Be mindful of the fact that Christmas trees do *not* decorate themselves—meaning, be thankful for others who have already invested time in you!

If tonight was the night before Christmas and it were your time to shine, would you be ready to be put on display? What if you were a Christmas tree and tomorrow was Christmas day?

FROM THE AUTHOR

The details of our lives are like the tiny individual brush strokes on a canvas. Those seemingly insignificant brush strokes can someday be viewed collectively as a valuable work of art!

Change tomorrow's poor health outcomes by reshaping your attitude and actions toward better health today!

According to the National Library of Medicine, in 1966 a forty-year longitudinal bed-rest study was performed on five twenty-year-old healthy males at Parkland Hospital in Dallas, Texas.

This is an important note because a forty-year study launched in 1966 would not conclude until 2006. By the time the researchers reached their findings, I was forty years old!

By age 40, it occurred to me that my purpose is to help healthy people stay healthy!

My goal was to master the subject of being well. The wellness industry took me to places I'd only dreamed about as a child. I wanted to appear on TV, radio, newspapers, and magazines. Not for personal fame or fortune. Rather, I wanted an opportunity to inspire others to be well! I wanted to be the spark that made people get up and do *something* about their lives to make life a little more *meaningful*. I've always believed that anything worth having is worth putting in the necessary time and effort.

My health journey started in 1971. I was five years old watching my favorite television show, *The Jack Lalanne Show*.

The Jack Lalanne Show was an exercise TV show hosted by nutritionist and author Jack Lalanne.

Jack's opening statement was always, "I want you to look better and feel better so that you can live longer."

Jack always appeared energetic, sincere, and enthusiastic about helping people live a healthy life!

I wanted to someday become the next Jack Lalanne!

Jack had no idea that I would be glued to my little thirteen-inch black-and-white television screen over fifty years ago as a Jack Lalanne intern!

Like Jack, I wanted to carve out a powerful message to share with others. Powerful messages are like good music; it has a way of finding its audiences.

Don't look for the quickest, easiest weight loss plan. Look for more sustainable, healthier solutions.

I've always believed that fitness is the ultimate *"want to"* business, because it is still one of the few things in life you have to earn. For more than two decades, I've witnessed people transform themselves from, the seemingly hopeless to, the invincible!

NOTES AND ANALYSIS REVIEW

1. How many days per week do you exercise?
2. How many days per week do you eat meals you did not prepare?
3. What are your unhealthy habits?
4. What are your healthier habits?
5. What is your immediate goal?
6. What will be the result after achieving your immediate goal?
7. What's the difference between goals and results?
8. Before reading this study guide, was your attitude positive or negative about diet and exercise?
9. How much has my *FATMAP Study Guide* changed your attitude?
10. After reading this study guide, do you feel more or less in control of your health?
11. In which area do you need more assistance, diet or exercise?
12. Do you want to lose or gain weight?
13. How do you tell your body to gain or lose weight?
14. True or false: Exercise makes you lose weight?
15. True or false: Your weight is one number?
16. What are the three eating components to weight control?
17. Do you want to build muscle?
18. Do you want to lose body fat?
19. Do you need to develop more strength and stamina?
20. Do you need more energy?
21. What do you need to change in order to achieve better health?
22. What is meant by "good health is not purchased?"
23. What's more important, avoiding calories or food chemicals?

24. What is meant by the "gift of good health?"
25. Which should you focus on, goals or results?
26. What's the difference between long-term and ultimate goal?
27. What's the first thing you should do before starting your workouts?

Physical Activity Readiness Questionnaire (PAR-Q)

28. Has a doctor ever said you have a heart condition and recommended only medically supervised physical activity?
29. Do you have chest pain brought on by physical activity?
30. Have you experienced low back pain in the past six months?
31. Do you lose consciousness or fall over as a result of dizziness?
32. Are you currently pregnant, or have you given birth within the past six months?
33. Has a doctor ever recommended medication for your blood pressure or heart condition?
34. Do you have a bone or joint problem that could be aggravated by physical activity?
35. Are you aware of any reason preventing you from exercise without medical supervision?
36. Are you over the age of sixty-five and are not accustomed to vigorous exercise?
37. Have you been diagnosed with a compulsive overeating disorder?
38. Do you have food allergies, or are you currently on a medically supervised special diet?
39. Have you consulted your physician regarding dietary changes or increasing your physical activity?

Before starting my FATMAP program, please consider questions 28-39.

FATMAP Step-by-Step Helpful Tips

Study your notes and prepare your food ahead of time. Store your food and supplements in a place convenient for quick consumption. This is crucial!

Step 1: Keep a food log for ten to fourteen days prior to starting my FATMAP Program.

Step 2: Order supplements (optional). For more information about supplements, please visit myj42.com or firstfitnessnutrition.com.

Step 3: Create a 20/20 foods list. The 20/20 list contains twenty healthy foods you will eat and twenty unhealthy foods you would normally eat but will avoid.

Step 4: Write down your start weight and waistline around your belly button. Please include your start date.

Step 5: Prepare your meals one to two days before starting.

A good practice is to blend or mix the meat protein with your vegetables.

Keys to Success

- Focus on food you are allowed to eat.
- Use natural seasonings (peppers, onions, etc.).
- Separate food into convenient, portable containers.

Phase 1: Elimination Phase, Day 1–7

- Weight loss starts with regular daily trips to the restroom dispelling waste that would otherwise be stored in your body.
- Your complete health involves replacing acidic foods with foods that are more alkaline.
- Speed up digestion by eating less dense foods.

- Eat whole foods that are quickly eliminated.

Do not eat from the following list for the first seven days:

- Fried food
- Fast food
- Shellfish
- Catfish
- Pork
- Breaded meat
- Processed hot dogs and lunch meats
- Dairy products
- Soft drinks
- Alcoholic beverages

Note:
Stick to one six- to eight-ounce lean meat per day. For example,

a. eat only fish protein on day 1,
b. eat only chicken protein on day 2.
c. eat only beef protein on day 3,
d. eat unlimited fresh or frozen vegetables daily.

Phase 1 lasts seven days.

Phase 2: Day 8–22

Phase 2 lasts fourteen days.

- Bring over everything from phase 1.
- Add low acidic and low glycemic food.
- Search glycemic index.
- Update weight and waistline measurements on day 8.

Phase 3: Day 23–42

- Update weight and waistline measurements on days 23 and 42.
- Add low-density foods. Low-density foods are low calorie.
- Energy density drives weight
- Vegetables are low density
- High density is small servings with high calories like chips and candy.

RESOURCES

Amen, Daniel G. *Change Your Brain Change Your Life*. New York, NY: Member of The Crown Publishing Group, 1998.

Lavelle, James B. *Cracking the Metabolic Code*. North Bergen, NJ: Basic Health Publications Inc., 2004.

Baillie-Hamilton, Paula. *Toxic Overload. A Doctor's Plan for Combating the Illnesses Caused by Chemicals in Our Foods Our Homes, and Our Medicine Cabinets*. New York, NY: The Penguin Group. 2005.

Davis, William. *Wheat Belly*. New York, NY: Royale Inc., 2011.

Doidge, Norman. *The Brain That Changes Itself*. Strand, London: Penguin Books, 2007.

Nestle, Marion. *Food Politics*. London, England: University of California Press, 2002.

Pilzer, Paul Zane. *The New Wellness Revolution*, 2nd ed. Hoboken, New Jersey: John Wiley & Sons, Inc., 2002, 2007.

ABOUT THE AUTHOR

Gerald Keith Jackson is a national certified personal trainer and certified dietary guidance consultant who provides an in-depth presentation on the benefits of adopting a comprehensive approach to health and wellness.

Gerald has developed the FATMAP program, which he shares with his audiences.

Gerald is a dynamic speaker and master motivator who inspires his audience to take charge of their well-being. His passion is helping others reach their goals and live their happiest, healthiest, most fulfilling life.

Gerald has over twenty years of professional experience successfully transforming people into healthier, more disciplined individuals.

He has nationally published fitness articles in over thirty-six states since 2007.

According to Gerald, "A negative thought is the most weight you will ever lift."

www.ingramcontent.com/pod-product-compliance
Lightning Source LLC
Chambersburg PA
CBHW051333150726

47997CB00004B/1446